NURSING
PHARMACOLOGY
NOTEBOOK

_____

_____

_____

_____

GENERIC NAME	DRUG CLASS
TRADE NAME	HIGH ALERT: YES/NO

Mechanism of Action:	Therapeutic Uses:	Contraindications:

Adverse Reaction/ Side Effects:	Nursing Considerations:	Patient Education:

NOTES:

GENERIC NAME	DRUG CLASS
TRADE NAME	HIGH ALERT: YES/NO

Mechanism of Action:	Therapeutic Uses:	Contraindications:

Adverse Reaction/ Side Effects:	Nursing Considerations:	Patient Education:

NOTES:

GENERIC NAME	DRUG CLASS
TRADE NAME	HIGH ALERT: YES/NO

Mechanism of Action:	Therapeutic Uses:	Contraindications:

Adverse Reaction/ Side Effects:	Nursing Considerations:	Patient Education:

NOTES:

GENERIC NAME	DRUG CLASS
TRADE NAME	HIGH ALERT: YES/NO

Mechanism of Action:	Therapeutic Uses:	Contraindications:

Adverse Reaction/ Side Effects:	Nursing Considerations:	Patient Education:

NOTES:

GENERIC NAME	DRUG CLASS
TRADE NAME	HIGH ALERT: YES/NO

Mechanism of Action:

Therapeutic Uses:

Contraindications:

Adverse Reaction/ Side Effects:

Nursing Considerations:

Patient Education:

NOTES:

GENERIC NAME	DRUG CLASS
TRADE NAME	HIGH ALERT: YES/NO

Mechanism of Action:	Therapeutic Uses:	Contraindications:

Adverse Reaction/ Side Effects:	Nursing Considerations:	Patient Education:

NOTES:

GENERIC NAME	DRUG CLASS
TRADE NAME	HIGH ALERT: YES/NO

Mechanism of Action:

Therapeutic Uses:

Contraindications:

Adverse Reaction/ Side Effects:

Nursing Considerations:

Patient Education:

NOTES:

GENERIC NAME	DRUG CLASS
TRADE NAME	HIGH ALERT: YES/NO

Mechanism of Action:	Therapeutic Uses:	Contraindications:

Adverse Reaction/ Side Effects:	Nursing Considerations:	Patient Education:

NOTES:

GENERIC NAME	DRUG CLASS
TRADE NAME	HIGH ALERT: YES/NO

Mechanism of Action:

Therapeutic Uses:

Contraindications:

Adverse Reaction/ Side Effects:

Nursing Considerations:

Patient Education:

NOTES:

GENERIC NAME	DRUG CLASS
TRADE NAME	HIGH ALERT: YES/NO

Mechanism of Action:	Therapeutic Uses:	Contraindications:

Adverse Reaction/ Side Effects:	Nursing Considerations:	Patient Education:

NOTES:

GENERIC NAME	DRUG CLASS
TRADE NAME	HIGH ALERT: YES/NO

Mechanism of Action:

Therapeutic Uses:

Contraindications:

Adverse Reaction/
Side Effects:

Nursing
Considerations:

Patient Education:

NOTES:

GENERIC NAME	DRUG CLASS
TRADE NAME	HIGH ALERT: YES/NO

Mechanism of Action:	Therapeutic Uses:	Contraindications:

Adverse Reaction/ Side Effects:	Nursing Considerations:	Patient Education:

NOTES:

GENERIC NAME	DRUG CLASS
TRADE NAME	HIGH ALERT: YES/NO

Mechanism of Action:	Therapeutic Uses:	Contraindications:

Adverse Reaction/ Side Effects:	Nursing Considerations:	Patient Education:

NOTES:

GENERIC NAME	DRUG CLASS
TRADE NAME	HIGH ALERT: YES/NO

Mechanism of Action:

Therapeutic Uses:

Contraindications:

Adverse Reaction/
Side Effects:

Nursing
Considerations:

Patient Education:

NOTES:

GENERIC NAME	DRUG CLASS
TRADE NAME	HIGH ALERT: YES/NO

Mechanism of Action:	Therapeutic Uses:	Contraindications:

Adverse Reaction/ Side Effects:	Nursing Considerations:	Patient Education:

NOTES:

GENERIC NAME	DRUG CLASS
TRADE NAME	HIGH ALERT: YES/NO

Mechanism of Action:

Therapeutic Uses:

Contraindications:

Adverse Reaction/ Side Effects:

Nursing Considerations:

Patient Education:

NOTES:

GENERIC NAME	DRUG CLASS
TRADE NAME	HIGH ALERT: YES/NO

Mechanism of Action:

Therapeutic Uses:

Contraindications:

Adverse Reaction/
Side Effects:

Nursing
Considerations:

Patient Education:

NOTES:

GENERIC NAME	DRUG CLASS
TRADE NAME	HIGH ALERT: YES/NO

Mechanism of Action:	Therapeutic Uses:	Contraindications:

Adverse Reaction/ Side Effects:	Nursing Considerations:	Patient Education:

NOTES:

GENERIC NAME	DRUG CLASS
TRADE NAME	HIGH ALERT: YES/NO

Mechanism of Action:	Therapeutic Uses:	Contraindications:

Adverse Reaction/ Side Effects:	Nursing Considerations:	Patient Education:

NOTES:

GENERIC NAME	DRUG CLASS
TRADE NAME	HIGH ALERT: YES/NO

Mechanism of Action:

Therapeutic Uses:

Contraindications:

Adverse Reaction/
Side Effects:

Nursing
Considerations:

Patient Education:

NOTES:

GENERIC NAME	DRUG CLASS
TRADE NAME	HIGH ALERT: YES/NO

Mechanism of Action:

Therapeutic Uses:

Contraindications:

Adverse Reaction/ Side Effects:

Nursing Considerations:

Patient Education:

NOTES:

GENERIC NAME	DRUG CLASS
TRADE NAME	HIGH ALERT: YES/NO

Mechanism of Action:	Therapeutic Uses:	Contraindications:

Adverse Reaction/ Side Effects:	Nursing Considerations:	Patient Education:

NOTES:

GENERIC NAME	DRUG CLASS
TRADE NAME	HIGH ALERT: YES/NO

Mechanism of Action:

Therapeutic Uses:

Contraindications:

Adverse Reaction/ Side Effects:

Nursing Considerations:

Patient Education:

NOTES:

GENERIC NAME	DRUG CLASS
TRADE NAME	HIGH ALERT: YES/NO

Mechanism of Action:	Therapeutic Uses:	Contraindications:

Adverse Reaction/ Side Effects:	Nursing Considerations:	Patient Education:

NOTES:

GENERIC NAME	DRUG CLASS
TRADE NAME	HIGH ALERT: YES/NO

Mechanism of Action:	Therapeutic Uses:	Contraindications:

Adverse Reaction/ Side Effects:	Nursing Considerations:	Patient Education:

NOTES:

GENERIC NAME	DRUG CLASS
TRADE NAME	HIGH ALERT: YES/NO

Mechanism of Action:	Therapeutic Uses:	Contraindications:

Adverse Reaction/ Side Effects:	Nursing Considerations:	Patient Education:

NOTES:

GENERIC NAME	DRUG CLASS
TRADE NAME	HIGH ALERT: YES/NO

Mechanism of Action:	Therapeutic Uses:	Contraindications:

Adverse Reaction/ Side Effects:	Nursing Considerations:	Patient Education:

NOTES:

GENERIC NAME	DRUG CLASS
TRADE NAME	HIGH ALERT: YES/NO

Mechanism of Action:

Therapeutic Uses:

Contraindications:

Adverse Reaction/ Side Effects:

Nursing Considerations:

Patient Education:

NOTES:

GENERIC NAME	DRUG CLASS
TRADE NAME	HIGH ALERT: YES/NO

Mechanism of Action:

Therapeutic Uses:

Contraindications:

Adverse Reaction/
Side Effects:

Nursing
Considerations:

Patient Education:

NOTES:

GENERIC NAME	DRUG CLASS
TRADE NAME	HIGH ALERT: YES/NO

Mechanism of Action:

Therapeutic Uses:

Contraindications:

Adverse Reaction/ Side Effects:

Nursing Considerations:

Patient Education:

NOTES:

GENERIC NAME	DRUG CLASS
TRADE NAME	HIGH ALERT: YES/NO

Mechanism of Action:	Therapeutic Uses:	Contraindications:

Adverse Reaction/ Side Effects:	Nursing Considerations:	Patient Education:

NOTES:

GENERIC NAME	DRUG CLASS
TRADE NAME	HIGH ALERT: YES/NO

Mechanism of Action:	Therapeutic Uses:	Contraindications:

Adverse Reaction/ Side Effects:	Nursing Considerations:	Patient Education:

NOTES:

GENERIC NAME	DRUG CLASS
TRADE NAME	HIGH ALERT: YES/NO

Mechanism of Action:

Therapeutic Uses:

Contraindications:

Adverse Reaction/ Side Effects:

Nursing Considerations:

Patient Education:

NOTES:

GENERIC NAME	DRUG CLASS
TRADE NAME	HIGH ALERT: YES/NO

Mechanism of Action:	Therapeutic Uses:	Contraindications:

Adverse Reaction/ Side Effects:	Nursing Considerations:	Patient Education:

NOTES:

GENERIC NAME	DRUG CLASS
TRADE NAME	HIGH ALERT: YES/NO

Mechanism of Action:

Therapeutic Uses:

Contraindications:

Adverse Reaction/
Side Effects:

Nursing
Considerations:

Patient Education:

NOTES:

GENERIC NAME	DRUG CLASS
TRADE NAME	HIGH ALERT: YES/NO

Mechanism of Action:

Therapeutic Uses:

Contraindications:

Adverse Reaction/ Side Effects:

Nursing Considerations:

Patient Education:

NOTES:

GENERIC NAME	DRUG CLASS
TRADE NAME	HIGH ALERT: YES/NO

Mechanism of Action:

Therapeutic Uses:

Contraindications:

Adverse Reaction/ Side Effects:

Nursing Considerations:

Patient Education:

NOTES:

GENERIC NAME	DRUG CLASS
TRADE NAME	HIGH ALERT: YES/NO

Mechanism of Action:	Therapeutic Uses:	Contraindications:

Adverse Reaction/ Side Effects:	Nursing Considerations:	Patient Education:

NOTES:

GENERIC NAME	DRUG CLASS
TRADE NAME	HIGH ALERT: YES/NO

Mechanism of Action:	Therapeutic Uses:	Contraindications:

Adverse Reaction/ Side Effects:	Nursing Considerations:	Patient Education:

NOTES:

GENERIC NAME	DRUG CLASS
TRADE NAME	HIGH ALERT: YES/NO

Mechanism of Action:	Therapeutic Uses:	Contraindications:

Adverse Reaction/ Side Effects:	Nursing Considerations:	Patient Education:

NOTES:

GENERIC NAME	DRUG CLASS
TRADE NAME	HIGH ALERT: YES/NO

Mechanism of Action:	Therapeutic Uses:	Contraindications:

Adverse Reaction/ Side Effects:	Nursing Considerations:	Patient Education:

NOTES:

GENERIC NAME	DRUG CLASS
TRADE NAME	HIGH ALERT: YES/NO

Mechanism of Action:	Therapeutic Uses:	Contraindications:

Adverse Reaction/ Side Effects:	Nursing Considerations:	Patient Education:

NOTES:

GENERIC NAME	DRUG CLASS
TRADE NAME	HIGH ALERT: YES/NO

Mechanism of Action:	Therapeutic Uses:	Contraindications:

Adverse Reaction/ Side Effects:	Nursing Considerations:	Patient Education:

NOTES:

GENERIC NAME	DRUG CLASS
TRADE NAME	HIGH ALERT: YES/NO

Mechanism of Action:

Therapeutic Uses:

Contraindications:

Adverse Reaction/ Side Effects:

Nursing Considerations:

Patient Education:

NOTES:

GENERIC NAME	DRUG CLASS
TRADE NAME	HIGH ALERT: YES/NO

Mechanism of Action:

Therapeutic Uses:

Contraindications:

Adverse Reaction/ Side Effects:

Nursing Considerations:

Patient Education:

NOTES:

GENERIC NAME	DRUG CLASS
TRADE NAME	HIGH ALERT: YES/NO

Mechanism of Action:	Therapeutic Uses:	Contraindications:

Adverse Reaction/ Side Effects:	Nursing Considerations:	Patient Education:

NOTES:

GENERIC NAME	DRUG CLASS
TRADE NAME	HIGH ALERT: YES/NO

Mechanism of Action:	Therapeutic Uses:	Contraindications:

Adverse Reaction/ Side Effects:	Nursing Considerations:	Patient Education:

NOTES:

GENERIC NAME	DRUG CLASS
TRADE NAME	HIGH ALERT: YES/NO

Mechanism of Action:	Therapeutic Uses:	Contraindications:

Adverse Reaction/ Side Effects:	Nursing Considerations:	Patient Education:

NOTES:

GENERIC NAME	DRUG CLASS
TRADE NAME	HIGH ALERT: YES/NO

Mechanism of Action:

Therapeutic Uses:

Contraindications:

Adverse Reaction/ Side Effects:

Nursing Considerations:

Patient Education:

NOTES:

GENERIC NAME	DRUG CLASS
TRADE NAME	HIGH ALERT: YES/NO

Mechanism of Action:

Therapeutic Uses:

Contraindications:

Adverse Reaction/ Side Effects:

Nursing Considerations:

Patient Education:

NOTES:

GENERIC NAME

DRUG CLASS

TRADE NAME

HIGH ALERT: YES/NO

Mechanism of Action:

Therapeutic Uses:

Contraindications:

Adverse Reaction/
Side Effects:

Nursing
Considerations:

Patient Education:

NOTES:

GENERIC NAME	DRUG CLASS
TRADE NAME	HIGH ALERT: YES/NO

Mechanism of Action:

Therapeutic Uses:

Contraindications:

Adverse Reaction/
Side Effects:

Nursing
Considerations:

Patient Education:

NOTES:

GENERIC NAME	DRUG CLASS
TRADE NAME	HIGH ALERT: YES/NO

Mechanism of Action:	Therapeutic Uses:	Contraindications:

Adverse Reaction/ Side Effects:	Nursing Considerations:	Patient Education:

NOTES:

GENERIC NAME	DRUG CLASS
TRADE NAME	HIGH ALERT: YES/NO

Mechanism of Action:	Therapeutic Uses:	Contraindications:

Adverse Reaction/ Side Effects:	Nursing Considerations:	Patient Education:

NOTES:

GENERIC NAME	DRUG CLASS
TRADE NAME	HIGH ALERT: YES/NO

Mechanism of Action:	Therapeutic Uses:	Contraindications:

Adverse Reaction/ Side Effects:	Nursing Considerations:	Patient Education:

NOTES:

GENERIC NAME	DRUG CLASS
TRADE NAME	HIGH ALERT: YES/NO

Mechanism of Action:	Therapeutic Uses:	Contraindications:

Adverse Reaction/ Side Effects:	Nursing Considerations:	Patient Education:

NOTES:

GENERIC NAME	DRUG CLASS
TRADE NAME	HIGH ALERT: YES/NO

Mechanism of Action:	Therapeutic Uses:	Contraindications:

Adverse Reaction/ Side Effects:	Nursing Considerations:	Patient Education:

NOTES:

GENERIC NAME	DRUG CLASS
TRADE NAME	HIGH ALERT: YES/NO

Mechanism of Action:

Therapeutic Uses:

Contraindications:

Adverse Reaction/ Side Effects:

Nursing Considerations:

Patient Education:

NOTES:

GENERIC NAME	DRUG CLASS
TRADE NAME	HIGH ALERT: YES/NO

Mechanism of Action:

Therapeutic Uses:

Contraindications:

Adverse Reaction/ Side Effects:

Nursing Considerations:

Patient Education:

NOTES:

GENERIC NAME	DRUG CLASS
TRADE NAME	HIGH ALERT: YES/NO

Mechanism of Action:	Therapeutic Uses:	Contraindications:

Adverse Reaction/ Side Effects:	Nursing Considerations:	Patient Education:

NOTES:

GENERIC NAME	DRUG CLASS
TRADE NAME	HIGH ALERT: YES/NO

Mechanism of Action:	Therapeutic Uses:	Contraindications:

Adverse Reaction/ Side Effects:	Nursing Considerations:	Patient Education:

NOTES:

GENERIC NAME	DRUG CLASS
TRADE NAME	HIGH ALERT: YES/NO

Mechanism of Action:

Therapeutic Uses:

Contraindications:

Adverse Reaction/
Side Effects:

Nursing
Considerations:

Patient Education:

NOTES:

GENERIC NAME	DRUG CLASS
TRADE NAME	HIGH ALERT: YES/NO

Mechanism of Action:

Therapeutic Uses:

Contraindications:

Adverse Reaction/ Side Effects:

Nursing Considerations:

Patient Education:

NOTES:

GENERIC NAME	DRUG CLASS
TRADE NAME	HIGH ALERT: YES/NO

Mechanism of Action:	Therapeutic Uses:	Contraindications:

Adverse Reaction/ Side Effects:	Nursing Considerations:	Patient Education:

NOTES:

GENERIC NAME	DRUG CLASS
TRADE NAME	HIGH ALERT: YES/NO

Mechanism of Action:	Therapeutic Uses:	Contraindications:

Adverse Reaction/ Side Effects:	Nursing Considerations:	Patient Education:

NOTES:

GENERIC NAME	DRUG CLASS
TRADE NAME	HIGH ALERT: YES/NO

Mechanism of Action:	Therapeutic Uses:	Contraindications:

Adverse Reaction/ Side Effects:	Nursing Considerations:	Patient Education:

NOTES:

GENERIC NAME	DRUG CLASS
TRADE NAME	HIGH ALERT: YES/NO

Mechanism of Action:	Therapeutic Uses:	Contraindications:

Adverse Reaction/ Side Effects:	Nursing Considerations:	Patient Education:

NOTES:

GENERIC NAME	DRUG CLASS
TRADE NAME	HIGH ALERT: YES/NO

Mechanism of Action:	Therapeutic Uses:	Contraindications:

Adverse Reaction/ Side Effects:	Nursing Considerations:	Patient Education:

NOTES:

GENERIC NAME	DRUG CLASS
TRADE NAME	HIGH ALERT: YES/NO

Mechanism of Action:	Therapeutic Uses:	Contraindications:

Adverse Reaction/ Side Effects:	Nursing Considerations:	Patient Education:

NOTES:

GENERIC NAME	DRUG CLASS
TRADE NAME	HIGH ALERT: YES/NO

Mechanism of Action:

Therapeutic Uses:

Contraindications:

Adverse Reaction/ Side Effects:

Nursing Considerations:

Patient Education:

NOTES:

GENERIC NAME	DRUG CLASS
TRADE NAME	HIGH ALERT: YES/NO

Mechanism of Action:	Therapeutic Uses:	Contraindications:

Adverse Reaction/ Side Effects:	Nursing Considerations:	Patient Education:

NOTES:

GENERIC NAME	DRUG CLASS
TRADE NAME	HIGH ALERT: YES/NO

Mechanism of Action:	Therapeutic Uses:	Contraindications:

Adverse Reaction/ Side Effects:	Nursing Considerations:	Patient Education:

NOTES:

GENERIC NAME	DRUG CLASS
TRADE NAME	HIGH ALERT: YES/NO

Mechanism of Action:	Therapeutic Uses:	Contraindications:

Adverse Reaction/ Side Effects:	Nursing Considerations:	Patient Education:

NOTES:

GENERIC NAME	DRUG CLASS
TRADE NAME	HIGH ALERT: YES/NO

Mechanism of Action:	Therapeutic Uses:	Contraindications:

Adverse Reaction/ Side Effects:	Nursing Considerations:	Patient Education:

NOTES:

GENERIC NAME

TRADE NAME

DRUG CLASS

HIGH ALERT: YES/NO

Mechanism of Action:

Therapeutic Uses:

Contraindications:

Adverse Reaction/
Side Effects:

Nursing
Considerations:

Patient Education:

NOTES:

GENERIC NAME	DRUG CLASS
TRADE NAME	HIGH ALERT: YES/NO

Mechanism of Action:

Therapeutic Uses:

Contraindications:

Adverse Reaction/
Side Effects:

Nursing
Considerations:

Patient Education:

NOTES:

GENERIC NAME	DRUG CLASS
TRADE NAME	HIGH ALERT: YES/NO

Mechanism of Action:	Therapeutic Uses:	Contraindications:

Adverse Reaction/ Side Effects:	Nursing Considerations:	Patient Education:

NOTES:

GENERIC NAME	DRUG CLASS
TRADE NAME	HIGH ALERT: YES/NO

Mechanism of Action:	Therapeutic Uses:	Contraindications:

Adverse Reaction/ Side Effects:	Nursing Considerations:	Patient Education:

NOTES:

GENERIC NAME	DRUG CLASS
TRADE NAME	HIGH ALERT: YES/NO

Mechanism of Action:	Therapeutic Uses:	Contraindications:

Adverse Reaction/ Side Effects:	Nursing Considerations:	Patient Education:

NOTES:

GENERIC NAME	DRUG CLASS
TRADE NAME	HIGH ALERT: YES/NO

Mechanism of Action:

Therapeutic Uses:

Contraindications:

Adverse Reaction/ Side Effects:

Nursing Considerations:

Patient Education:

NOTES:

GENERIC NAME	DRUG CLASS
TRADE NAME	HIGH ALERT: YES/NO

Mechanism of Action:	Therapeutic Uses:	Contraindications:

Adverse Reaction/ Side Effects:	Nursing Considerations:	Patient Education:

NOTES:

GENERIC NAME

DRUG CLASS

TRADE NAME

HIGH ALERT: YES/NO

Mechanism of Action:

Therapeutic Uses:

Contraindications:

Adverse Reaction/
Side Effects:

Nursing
Considerations:

Patient Education:

NOTES:

GENERIC NAME	DRUG CLASS
TRADE NAME	HIGH ALERT: YES/NO

Mechanism of Action:	Therapeutic Uses:	Contraindications:

Adverse Reaction/ Side Effects:	Nursing Considerations:	Patient Education:

NOTES:

GENERIC NAME	DRUG CLASS
TRADE NAME	HIGH ALERT: YES/NO

Mechanism of Action:

Therapeutic Uses:

Contraindications:

Adverse Reaction/ Side Effects:

Nursing Considerations:

Patient Education:

NOTES:

GENERIC NAME	DRUG CLASS
TRADE NAME	HIGH ALERT: YES/NO

Mechanism of Action:	Therapeutic Uses:	Contraindications:

Adverse Reaction/ Side Effects:	Nursing Considerations:	Patient Education:

NOTES:

GENERIC NAME	DRUG CLASS
TRADE NAME	HIGH ALERT: YES/NO

Mechanism of Action:	Therapeutic Uses:	Contraindications:

Adverse Reaction/ Side Effects:	Nursing Considerations:	Patient Education:

NOTES:

GENERIC NAME	DRUG CLASS
TRADE NAME	HIGH ALERT: YES/NO

Mechanism of Action:	Therapeutic Uses:	Contraindications:

Adverse Reaction/ Side Effects:	Nursing Considerations:	Patient Education:

NOTES:

GENERIC NAME	DRUG CLASS
TRADE NAME	HIGH ALERT: YES/NO

Mechanism of Action:

Therapeutic Uses:

Contraindications:

Adverse Reaction/ Side Effects:

Nursing Considerations:

Patient Education:

NOTES:

GENERIC NAME	DRUG CLASS
TRADE NAME	HIGH ALERT: YES/NO

Mechanism of Action:	Therapeutic Uses:	Contraindications:

Adverse Reaction/ Side Effects:	Nursing Considerations:	Patient Education:

NOTES:

GENERIC NAME	DRUG CLASS
TRADE NAME	HIGH ALERT: YES/NO

Mechanism of Action:

Therapeutic Uses:

Contraindications:

Adverse Reaction/ Side Effects:

Nursing Considerations:

Patient Education:

NOTES:

GENERIC NAME	DRUG CLASS
TRADE NAME	HIGH ALERT: YES/NO

Mechanism of Action:	Therapeutic Uses:	Contraindications:

Adverse Reaction/ Side Effects:	Nursing Considerations:	Patient Education:

NOTES:

GENERIC NAME	DRUG CLASS
TRADE NAME	HIGH ALERT: YES/NO

Mechanism of Action:	Therapeutic Uses:	Contraindications:

Adverse Reaction/ Side Effects:	Nursing Considerations:	Patient Education:

NOTES:

GENERIC NAME	DRUG CLASS
TRADE NAME	HIGH ALERT: YES/NO

Mechanism of Action:

Therapeutic Uses:

Contraindications:

Adverse Reaction/ Side Effects:

Nursing Considerations:

Patient Education:

NOTES:

GENERIC NAME	DRUG CLASS
TRADE NAME	HIGH ALERT: YES/NO

Mechanism of Action:

Therapeutic Uses:

Contraindications:

Adverse Reaction/ Side Effects:

Nursing Considerations:

Patient Education:

NOTES:

GENERIC NAME	DRUG CLASS
TRADE NAME	HIGH ALERT: YES/NO

Mechanism of Action:	Therapeutic Uses:	Contraindications:

Adverse Reaction/ Side Effects:	Nursing Considerations:	Patient Education:

NOTES:

GENERIC NAME	DRUG CLASS
TRADE NAME	HIGH ALERT: YES/NO

Mechanism of Action:	Therapeutic Uses:	Contraindications:

Adverse Reaction/ Side Effects:	Nursing Considerations:	Patient Education:

NOTES:

GENERIC NAME	DRUG CLASS
TRADE NAME	HIGH ALERT: YES/NO

Mechanism of Action:

Therapeutic Uses:

Contraindications:

Adverse Reaction/ Side Effects:

Nursing Considerations:

Patient Education:

NOTES:

GENERIC NAME	DRUG CLASS
TRADE NAME	HIGH ALERT: YES/NO

Mechanism of Action:	Therapeutic Uses:	Contraindications:

Adverse Reaction/ Side Effects:	Nursing Considerations:	Patient Education:

NOTES:

GENERIC NAME	DRUG CLASS
TRADE NAME	HIGH ALERT: YES/NO

Mechanism of Action:	Therapeutic Uses:	Contraindications:

Adverse Reaction/ Side Effects:	Nursing Considerations:	Patient Education:

NOTES:

GENERIC NAME	DRUG CLASS
TRADE NAME	HIGH ALERT: YES/NO

Mechanism of Action:	Therapeutic Uses:	Contraindications:

Adverse Reaction/ Side Effects:	Nursing Considerations:	Patient Education:

NOTES:

GENERIC NAME	DRUG CLASS
TRADE NAME	HIGH ALERT: YES/NO

Mechanism of Action:

Therapeutic Uses:

Contraindications:

Adverse Reaction/ Side Effects:

Nursing Considerations:

Patient Education:

NOTES:

GENERIC NAME	DRUG CLASS
TRADE NAME	HIGH ALERT: YES/NO

Mechanism of Action:	Therapeutic Uses:	Contraindications:

Adverse Reaction/ Side Effects:	Nursing Considerations:	Patient Education:

NOTES:

GENERIC NAME	DRUG CLASS
TRADE NAME	HIGH ALERT: YES/NO

Mechanism of Action:	Therapeutic Uses:	Contraindications:

Adverse Reaction/ Side Effects:	Nursing Considerations:	Patient Education:

NOTES:

GENERIC NAME	DRUG CLASS
TRADE NAME	HIGH ALERT: YES/NO

Mechanism of Action:	Therapeutic Uses:	Contraindications:

Adverse Reaction/ Side Effects:	Nursing Considerations:	Patient Education:

NOTES:

GENERIC NAME	DRUG CLASS
TRADE NAME	HIGH ALERT: YES/NO

Mechanism of Action:	Therapeutic Uses:	Contraindications:

Adverse Reaction/ Side Effects:	Nursing Considerations:	Patient Education:

NOTES:

GENERIC NAME	DRUG CLASS
TRADE NAME	HIGH ALERT: YES/NO

Mechanism of Action:

Therapeutic Uses:

Contraindications:

Adverse Reaction/ Side Effects:

Nursing Considerations:

Patient Education:

NOTES:

GENERIC NAME	DRUG CLASS
TRADE NAME	HIGH ALERT: YES/NO

Mechanism of Action:

Therapeutic Uses:

Contraindications:

Adverse Reaction/ Side Effects:

Nursing Considerations:

Patient Education:

NOTES:

GENERIC NAME	DRUG CLASS
TRADE NAME	HIGH ALERT: YES/NO

Mechanism of Action:	Therapeutic Uses:	Contraindications:

Adverse Reaction/ Side Effects:	Nursing Considerations:	Patient Education:

NOTES:

GENERIC NAME	DRUG CLASS
TRADE NAME	HIGH ALERT: YES/NO

Mechanism of Action:	Therapeutic Uses:	Contraindications:

Adverse Reaction/ Side Effects:	Nursing Considerations:	Patient Education:

NOTES:

GENERIC NAME	DRUG CLASS
TRADE NAME	HIGH ALERT: YES/NO

Mechanism of Action:	Therapeutic Uses:	Contraindications:

Adverse Reaction/ Side Effects:	Nursing Considerations:	Patient Education:

NOTES:

GENERIC NAME	DRUG CLASS
TRADE NAME	HIGH ALERT: YES/NO

Mechanism of Action:

Therapeutic Uses:

Contraindications:

Adverse Reaction/ Side Effects:

Nursing Considerations:

Patient Education:

NOTES:

GENERIC NAME	DRUG CLASS
TRADE NAME	HIGH ALERT: YES/NO

Mechanism of Action:	Therapeutic Uses:	Contraindications:

Adverse Reaction/ Side Effects:	Nursing Considerations:	Patient Education:

NOTES:

GENERIC NAME	DRUG CLASS
TRADE NAME	HIGH ALERT: YES/NO

Mechanism of Action:

Therapeutic Uses:

Contraindications:

Adverse Reaction/
Side Effects:

Nursing
Considerations:

Patient Education:

NOTES:

GENERIC NAME	DRUG CLASS
TRADE NAME	HIGH ALERT: YES/NO

Mechanism of Action:	Therapeutic Uses:	Contraindications:

Adverse Reaction/ Side Effects:	Nursing Considerations:	Patient Education:

NOTES:

GENERIC NAME	DRUG CLASS
TRADE NAME	HIGH ALERT: YES/NO

Mechanism of Action:	Therapeutic Uses:	Contraindications:

Adverse Reaction/ Side Effects:	Nursing Considerations:	Patient Education:

NOTES:

GENERIC NAME	DRUG CLASS
TRADE NAME	HIGH ALERT: YES/NO

Mechanism of Action:	Therapeutic Uses:	Contraindications:

Adverse Reaction/ Side Effects:	Nursing Considerations:	Patient Education:

NOTES:

GENERIC NAME	DRUG CLASS
TRADE NAME	HIGH ALERT: YES/NO

Mechanism of Action:	Therapeutic Uses:	Contraindications:

Adverse Reaction/ Side Effects:	Nursing Considerations:	Patient Education:

NOTES:

GENERIC NAME	DRUG CLASS
TRADE NAME	HIGH ALERT: YES/NO

Mechanism of Action:

Therapeutic Uses:

Contraindications:

Adverse Reaction/ Side Effects:

Nursing Considerations:

Patient Education:

NOTES:

GENERIC NAME	DRUG CLASS
TRADE NAME	HIGH ALERT: YES/NO

Mechanism of Action:

Therapeutic Uses:

Contraindications:

Adverse Reaction/ Side Effects:

Nursing Considerations:

Patient Education:

NOTES:

GENERIC NAME	DRUG CLASS
TRADE NAME	HIGH ALERT: YES/NO

Mechanism of Action:

Therapeutic Uses:

Contraindications:

Adverse Reaction/ Side Effects:

Nursing Considerations:

Patient Education:

NOTES:

GENERIC NAME	DRUG CLASS
TRADE NAME	HIGH ALERT: YES/NO

Mechanism of Action:	Therapeutic Uses:	Contraindications:

Adverse Reaction/ Side Effects:	Nursing Considerations:	Patient Education:

NOTES:

GENERIC NAME	DRUG CLASS
TRADE NAME	HIGH ALERT: YES/NO

Mechanism of Action:	Therapeutic Uses:	Contraindications:

Adverse Reaction/ Side Effects:	Nursing Considerations:	Patient Education:

NOTES:

GENERIC NAME	DRUG CLASS
TRADE NAME	HIGH ALERT: YES/NO

Mechanism of Action:	Therapeutic Uses:	Contraindications:

Adverse Reaction/ Side Effects:	Nursing Considerations:	Patient Education:

NOTES:

GENERIC NAME	DRUG CLASS
TRADE NAME	HIGH ALERT: YES/NO

Mechanism of Action:

Therapeutic Uses:

Contraindications:

Adverse Reaction/
Side Effects:

Nursing
Considerations:

Patient Education:

NOTES:

GENERIC NAME	DRUG CLASS
TRADE NAME	HIGH ALERT: YES/NO

Mechanism of Action:

Therapeutic Uses:

Contraindications:

Adverse Reaction/ Side Effects:

Nursing Considerations:

Patient Education:

NOTES:

GENERIC NAME	DRUG CLASS
TRADE NAME	HIGH ALERT: YES/NO

Mechanism of Action:

Therapeutic Uses:

Contraindications:

Adverse Reaction/ Side Effects:

Nursing Considerations:

Patient Education:

NOTES:

GENERIC NAME	DRUG CLASS
TRADE NAME	HIGH ALERT: YES/NO

Mechanism of Action:

Therapeutic Uses:

Contraindications:

Adverse Reaction/ Side Effects:

Nursing Considerations:

Patient Education:

NOTES:

GENERIC NAME	DRUG CLASS
TRADE NAME	HIGH ALERT: YES/NO

Mechanism of Action:

Therapeutic Uses:

Contraindications:

Adverse Reaction/ Side Effects:

Nursing Considerations:

Patient Education:

NOTES:

GENERIC NAME	DRUG CLASS
TRADE NAME	HIGH ALERT: YES/NO

Mechanism of Action:

Therapeutic Uses:

Contraindications:

Adverse Reaction/ Side Effects:

Nursing Considerations:

Patient Education:

NOTES:

GENERIC NAME	DRUG CLASS
TRADE NAME	HIGH ALERT: YES/NO

Mechanism of Action:	Therapeutic Uses:	Contraindications:

Adverse Reaction/ Side Effects:	Nursing Considerations:	Patient Education:

NOTES:

GENERIC NAME	DRUG CLASS
TRADE NAME	HIGH ALERT: YES/NO

Mechanism of Action:

Therapeutic Uses:

Contraindications:

Adverse Reaction/ Side Effects:

Nursing Considerations:

Patient Education:

NOTES:

GENERIC NAME	DRUG CLASS
TRADE NAME	HIGH ALERT: YES/NO

Mechanism of Action:

Therapeutic Uses:

Contraindications:

Adverse Reaction/ Side Effects:

Nursing Considerations:

Patient Education:

NOTES:

GENERIC NAME	DRUG CLASS
TRADE NAME	HIGH ALERT: YES/NO

Mechanism of Action:	Therapeutic Uses:	Contraindications:

Adverse Reaction/ Side Effects:	Nursing Considerations:	Patient Education:

NOTES:

GENERIC NAME	DRUG CLASS
TRADE NAME	HIGH ALERT: YES/NO

Mechanism of Action:	Therapeutic Uses:	Contraindications:

Adverse Reaction/ Side Effects:	Nursing Considerations:	Patient Education:

NOTES:

GENERIC NAME

DRUG CLASS

TRADE NAME

HIGH ALERT: YES/NO

Mechanism of Action:

Therapeutic Uses:

Contraindications:

Adverse Reaction/
Side Effects:

Nursing
Considerations:

Patient Education:

NOTES:

GENERIC NAME	DRUG CLASS
TRADE NAME	HIGH ALERT: YES/NO

Mechanism of Action:

Therapeutic Uses:

Contraindications:

Adverse Reaction/ Side Effects:

Nursing Considerations:

Patient Education:

NOTES:

GENERIC NAME	DRUG CLASS
TRADE NAME	HIGH ALERT: YES/NO

Mechanism of Action:

Therapeutic Uses:

Contraindications:

Adverse Reaction/ Side Effects:

Nursing Considerations:

Patient Education:

NOTES:

GENERIC NAME	DRUG CLASS
TRADE NAME	HIGH ALERT: YES/NO

Mechanism of Action:	Therapeutic Uses:	Contraindications:

Adverse Reaction/ Side Effects:	Nursing Considerations:	Patient Education:

NOTES:

GENERIC NAME	DRUG CLASS
TRADE NAME	HIGH ALERT: YES/NO

Mechanism of Action:	Therapeutic Uses:	Contraindications:

Adverse Reaction/ Side Effects:	Nursing Considerations:	Patient Education:

NOTES:

GENERIC NAME	DRUG CLASS
TRADE NAME	HIGH ALERT: YES/NO

Mechanism of Action:	Therapeutic Uses:	Contraindications:

Adverse Reaction/ Side Effects:	Nursing Considerations:	Patient Education:

NOTES:

GENERIC NAME	DRUG CLASS
TRADE NAME	HIGH ALERT: YES/NO

Mechanism of Action:

Therapeutic Uses:

Contraindications:

Adverse Reaction/ Side Effects:

Nursing Considerations:

Patient Education:

NOTES:

GENERIC NAME	DRUG CLASS
TRADE NAME	HIGH ALERT: YES/NO

Mechanism of Action:

Therapeutic Uses:

Contraindications:

Adverse Reaction/ Side Effects:

Nursing Considerations:

Patient Education:

NOTES:

GENERIC NAME	DRUG CLASS
TRADE NAME	HIGH ALERT: YES/NO

Mechanism of Action:	Therapeutic Uses:	Contraindications:

Adverse Reaction/ Side Effects:	Nursing Considerations:	Patient Education:

NOTES:

GENERIC NAME	DRUG CLASS
TRADE NAME	HIGH ALERT: YES/NO

Mechanism of Action:	Therapeutic Uses:	Contraindications:

Adverse Reaction/ Side Effects:	Nursing Considerations:	Patient Education:

NOTES:

GENERIC NAME	DRUG CLASS
TRADE NAME	HIGH ALERT: YES/NO

Mechanism of Action:	Therapeutic Uses:	Contraindications:

Adverse Reaction/ Side Effects:	Nursing Considerations:	Patient Education:

NOTES:

GENERIC NAME	DRUG CLASS
TRADE NAME	HIGH ALERT: YES/NO

Mechanism of Action:

Therapeutic Uses:

Contraindications:

Adverse Reaction/ Side Effects:

Nursing Considerations:

Patient Education:

NOTES:

GENERIC NAME	DRUG CLASS
TRADE NAME	HIGH ALERT: YES/NO

Mechanism of Action:	Therapeutic Uses:	Contraindications:

Adverse Reaction/ Side Effects:	Nursing Considerations:	Patient Education:

NOTES:

GENERIC NAME	DRUG CLASS
TRADE NAME	HIGH ALERT: YES/NO

Mechanism of Action:

Therapeutic Uses:

Contraindications:

Adverse Reaction/ Side Effects:

Nursing Considerations:

Patient Education:

NOTES:

GENERIC NAME	DRUG CLASS
TRADE NAME	HIGH ALERT: YES/NO

Mechanism of Action:

Therapeutic Uses:

Contraindications:

Adverse Reaction/ Side Effects:

Nursing Considerations:

Patient Education:

NOTES:

GENERIC NAME	DRUG CLASS
TRADE NAME	HIGH ALERT: YES/NO

Mechanism of Action:	Therapeutic Uses:	Contraindications:

Adverse Reaction/ Side Effects:	Nursing Considerations:	Patient Education:

NOTES:

GENERIC NAME	DRUG CLASS
TRADE NAME	HIGH ALERT: YES/NO

Mechanism of Action:	Therapeutic Uses:	Contraindications:

Adverse Reaction/ Side Effects:	Nursing Considerations:	Patient Education:

NOTES:

GENERIC NAME	DRUG CLASS
TRADE NAME	HIGH ALERT: YES/NO

Mechanism of Action:	Therapeutic Uses:	Contraindications:

Adverse Reaction/ Side Effects:	Nursing Considerations:	Patient Education:

NOTES:

GENERIC NAME	DRUG CLASS
TRADE NAME	HIGH ALERT: YES/NO

Mechanism of Action:	Therapeutic Uses:	Contraindications:

Adverse Reaction/ Side Effects:	Nursing Considerations:	Patient Education:

NOTES:

GENERIC NAME

TRADE NAME

DRUG CLASS

HIGH ALERT: YES/NO

Mechanism of Action:

Therapeutic Uses:

Contraindications:

Adverse Reaction/
Side Effects:

Nursing
Considerations:

Patient Education:

NOTES:

GENERIC NAME	DRUG CLASS
TRADE NAME	HIGH ALERT: YES/NO

Mechanism of Action:	Therapeutic Uses:	Contraindications:

Adverse Reaction/ Side Effects:	Nursing Considerations:	Patient Education:

NOTES:

GENERIC NAME	DRUG CLASS
TRADE NAME	HIGH ALERT: YES/NO

Mechanism of Action:	Therapeutic Uses:	Contraindications:

Adverse Reaction/ Side Effects:	Nursing Considerations:	Patient Education:

NOTES:

GENERIC NAME	DRUG CLASS
TRADE NAME	HIGH ALERT: YES/NO

Mechanism of Action:	Therapeutic Uses:	Contraindications:

Adverse Reaction/ Side Effects:	Nursing Considerations:	Patient Education:

NOTES:

GENERIC NAME	DRUG CLASS
TRADE NAME	HIGH ALERT: YES/NO

Mechanism of Action:	Therapeutic Uses:	Contraindications:

Adverse Reaction/ Side Effects:	Nursing Considerations:	Patient Education:

NOTES:

GENERIC NAME	DRUG CLASS
TRADE NAME	HIGH ALERT: YES/NO

Mechanism of Action:

Therapeutic Uses:

Contraindications:

Adverse Reaction/ Side Effects:

Nursing Considerations:

Patient Education:

NOTES:

| GENERIC NAME | DRUG CLASS |
| TRADE NAME | HIGH ALERT: YES/NO |

Mechanism of Action:

Therapeutic Uses:

Contraindications:

Adverse Reaction/ Side Effects:

Nursing Considerations:

Patient Education:

NOTES:

GENERIC NAME	DRUG CLASS
TRADE NAME	HIGH ALERT: YES/NO

Mechanism of Action:

Therapeutic Uses:

Contraindications:

Adverse Reaction/ Side Effects:

Nursing Considerations:

Patient Education:

NOTES:

GENERIC NAME	DRUG CLASS
TRADE NAME	HIGH ALERT: YES/NO

Mechanism of Action:

Therapeutic Uses:

Contraindications:

Adverse Reaction/ Side Effects:

Nursing Considerations:

Patient Education:

NOTES:

GENERIC NAME	DRUG CLASS
TRADE NAME	HIGH ALERT: YES/NO

Mechanism of Action:	Therapeutic Uses:	Contraindications:

Adverse Reaction/ Side Effects:	Nursing Considerations:	Patient Education:

NOTES:

GENERIC NAME	DRUG CLASS
TRADE NAME	HIGH ALERT: YES/NO

Mechanism of Action:	Therapeutic Uses:	Contraindications:

Adverse Reaction/ Side Effects:	Nursing Considerations:	Patient Education:

NOTES:

GENERIC NAME	DRUG CLASS
TRADE NAME	HIGH ALERT: YES/NO

Mechanism of Action:

Therapeutic Uses:

Contraindications:

Adverse Reaction/ Side Effects:

Nursing Considerations:

Patient Education:

NOTES:

GENERIC NAME	DRUG CLASS
TRADE NAME	HIGH ALERT: YES/NO

Mechanism of Action:

Therapeutic Uses:

Contraindications:

Adverse Reaction/
Side Effects:

Nursing
Considerations:

Patient Education:

NOTES:

GENERIC NAME	DRUG CLASS
TRADE NAME	HIGH ALERT: YES/NO

Mechanism of Action:

Therapeutic Uses:

Contraindications:

Adverse Reaction/ Side Effects:

Nursing Considerations:

Patient Education:

NOTES:

GENERIC NAME	DRUG CLASS
TRADE NAME	HIGH ALERT: YES/NO

Mechanism of Action:	Therapeutic Uses:	Contraindications:

Adverse Reaction/ Side Effects:	Nursing Considerations:	Patient Education:

NOTES:

GENERIC NAME	DRUG CLASS
TRADE NAME	HIGH ALERT: YES/NO

Mechanism of Action:	Therapeutic Uses:	Contraindications:

Adverse Reaction/ Side Effects:	Nursing Considerations:	Patient Education:

NOTES:

GENERIC NAME	DRUG CLASS
TRADE NAME	HIGH ALERT: YES/NO

Mechanism of Action:	Therapeutic Uses:	Contraindications:

Adverse Reaction/ Side Effects:	Nursing Considerations:	Patient Education:

NOTES:

GENERIC NAME	DRUG CLASS
TRADE NAME	HIGH ALERT: YES/NO

Mechanism of Action:	Therapeutic Uses:	Contraindications:

Adverse Reaction/ Side Effects:	Nursing Considerations:	Patient Education:

NOTES:

GENERIC NAME	DRUG CLASS
TRADE NAME	HIGH ALERT: YES/NO

Mechanism of Action:

Therapeutic Uses:

Contraindications:

Adverse Reaction/
Side Effects:

Nursing
Considerations:

Patient Education:

NOTES:

GENERIC NAME	DRUG CLASS
TRADE NAME	HIGH ALERT: YES/NO

Mechanism of Action:

Therapeutic Uses:

Contraindications:

Adverse Reaction/ Side Effects:

Nursing Considerations:

Patient Education:

NOTES:

GENERIC NAME	DRUG CLASS
TRADE NAME	HIGH ALERT: YES/NO

Mechanism of Action:	Therapeutic Uses:	Contraindications:

Adverse Reaction/ Side Effects:	Nursing Considerations:	Patient Education:

NOTES:

GENERIC NAME	DRUG CLASS
TRADE NAME	HIGH ALERT: YES/NO

Mechanism of Action:	Therapeutic Uses:	Contraindications:

Adverse Reaction/ Side Effects:	Nursing Considerations:	Patient Education:

NOTES:

GENERIC NAME	DRUG CLASS
TRADE NAME	HIGH ALERT: YES/NO

Mechanism of Action:

Therapeutic Uses:

Contraindications:

Adverse Reaction/ Side Effects:

Nursing Considerations:

Patient Education:

NOTES:

GENERIC NAME	DRUG CLASS
TRADE NAME	HIGH ALERT: YES/NO

Mechanism of Action:

Therapeutic Uses:

Contraindications:

Adverse Reaction/ Side Effects:

Nursing Considerations:

Patient Education:

NOTES:

GENERIC NAME	DRUG CLASS
TRADE NAME	HIGH ALERT: YES/NO

Mechanism of Action:

Therapeutic Uses:

Contraindications:

Adverse Reaction/ Side Effects:

Nursing Considerations:

Patient Education:

NOTES:

GENERIC NAME	DRUG CLASS
TRADE NAME	HIGH ALERT: YES/NO

Mechanism of Action:

Therapeutic Uses:

Contraindications:

Adverse Reaction/ Side Effects:

Nursing Considerations:

Patient Education:

NOTES:

GENERIC NAME	DRUG CLASS
TRADE NAME	HIGH ALERT: YES/NO

Mechanism of Action:	Therapeutic Uses:	Contraindications:

Adverse Reaction/ Side Effects:	Nursing Considerations:	Patient Education:

NOTES:

GENERIC NAME	DRUG CLASS
TRADE NAME	HIGH ALERT: YES/NO

Mechanism of Action:	Therapeutic Uses:	Contraindications:

Adverse Reaction/ Side Effects:	Nursing Considerations:	Patient Education:

NOTES:

GENERIC NAME	DRUG CLASS
TRADE NAME	HIGH ALERT: YES/NO

Mechanism of Action:	Therapeutic Uses:	Contraindications:

Adverse Reaction/ Side Effects:	Nursing Considerations:	Patient Education:

NOTES:

GENERIC NAME	DRUG CLASS
TRADE NAME	HIGH ALERT: YES/NO

Mechanism of Action:

Therapeutic Uses:

Contraindications:

Adverse Reaction/ Side Effects:

Nursing Considerations:

Patient Education:

NOTES:

GENERIC NAME	DRUG CLASS
TRADE NAME	HIGH ALERT: YES/NO

Mechanism of Action:

Therapeutic Uses:

Contraindications:

Adverse Reaction/
Side Effects:

Nursing
Considerations:

Patient Education:

NOTES:

GENERIC NAME	DRUG CLASS
TRADE NAME	HIGH ALERT: YES/NO

Mechanism of Action:	Therapeutic Uses:	Contraindications:

Adverse Reaction/ Side Effects:	Nursing Considerations:	Patient Education:

NOTES:

GENERIC NAME	DRUG CLASS
TRADE NAME	HIGH ALERT: YES/NO

Mechanism of Action:

Therapeutic Uses:

Contraindications:

Adverse Reaction/ Side Effects:

Nursing Considerations:

Patient Education:

NOTES:

GENERIC NAME	DRUG CLASS
TRADE NAME	HIGH ALERT: YES/NO

Mechanism of Action:	Therapeutic Uses:	Contraindications:

Adverse Reaction/ Side Effects:	Nursing Considerations:	Patient Education:

NOTES:

GENERIC NAME	DRUG CLASS
TRADE NAME	HIGH ALERT: YES/NO

Mechanism of Action:	Therapeutic Uses:	Contraindications:

Adverse Reaction/ Side Effects:	Nursing Considerations:	Patient Education:

NOTES:

GENERIC NAME	DRUG CLASS
TRADE NAME	HIGH ALERT: YES/NO

Mechanism of Action:	Therapeutic Uses:	Contraindications:

Adverse Reaction/ Side Effects:	Nursing Considerations:	Patient Education:

NOTES:

GENERIC NAME	DRUG CLASS
TRADE NAME	HIGH ALERT: YES/NO

Mechanism of Action:

Therapeutic Uses:

Contraindications:

Adverse Reaction/ Side Effects:

Nursing Considerations:

Patient Education:

NOTES:

GENERIC NAME	DRUG CLASS
TRADE NAME	HIGH ALERT: YES/NO

Mechanism of Action:

Therapeutic Uses:

Contraindications:

Adverse Reaction/ Side Effects:

Nursing Considerations:

Patient Education:

NOTES:

GENERIC NAME	DRUG CLASS
TRADE NAME	HIGH ALERT: YES/NO

Mechanism of Action:	Therapeutic Uses:	Contraindications:

Adverse Reaction/ Side Effects:	Nursing Considerations:	Patient Education:

NOTES:

GENERIC NAME	DRUG CLASS
TRADE NAME	HIGH ALERT: YES/NO

Mechanism of Action:	Therapeutic Uses:	Contraindications:

Adverse Reaction/ Side Effects:	Nursing Considerations:	Patient Education:

NOTES:

GENERIC NAME	DRUG CLASS
TRADE NAME	HIGH ALERT: YES/NO

Mechanism of Action:

Therapeutic Uses:

Contraindications:

Adverse Reaction/ Side Effects:

Nursing Considerations:

Patient Education:

NOTES:

GENERIC NAME	DRUG CLASS
TRADE NAME	HIGH ALERT: YES/NO

Mechanism of Action:	Therapeutic Uses:	Contraindications:

Adverse Reaction/ Side Effects:	Nursing Considerations:	Patient Education:

NOTES:

GENERIC NAME	DRUG CLASS
TRADE NAME	HIGH ALERT: YES/NO

Mechanism of Action:

Therapeutic Uses:

Contraindications:

Adverse Reaction/ Side Effects:

Nursing Considerations:

Patient Education:

NOTES:

GENERIC NAME	DRUG CLASS
TRADE NAME	HIGH ALERT: YES/NO

Mechanism of Action:	Therapeutic Uses:	Contraindications:

Adverse Reaction/ Side Effects:	Nursing Considerations:	Patient Education:

NOTES:

GENERIC NAME	DRUG CLASS
TRADE NAME	HIGH ALERT: YES/NO

Mechanism of Action:	Therapeutic Uses:	Contraindications:

Adverse Reaction/ Side Effects:	Nursing Considerations:	Patient Education:

NOTES:

GENERIC NAME	DRUG CLASS
TRADE NAME	HIGH ALERT: YES/NO

Mechanism of Action:	Therapeutic Uses:	Contraindications:

Adverse Reaction/ Side Effects:	Nursing Considerations:	Patient Education:

NOTES:

GENERIC NAME	DRUG CLASS
TRADE NAME	HIGH ALERT: YES/NO

Mechanism of Action:	Therapeutic Uses:	Contraindications:

Adverse Reaction/ Side Effects:	Nursing Considerations:	Patient Education:

NOTES:

NOTES

NOTES

NOTES

NOTES

NOTES

NOTES

NOTES

NOTES

Made in the USA
Coppell, TX
16 September 2021